THE COMPARATIVE ANATOMY OF MAN, THE HORSE, AND THE DOG

CONTAINING INFORMATION ON
SKELETONS, THE NERVOUS
SYSTEM AND OTHER ASPECTS
OF ANATOMY

PART IV

NATURAL HISTORY OF THE PRINCIPAL ANIMALS
USED BY MAN IN RURAL SPORTS

Copyright © 2013 Read Books Ltd.
This book is copyright and may not be
reproduced or copied in any way without
the express permission of the publisher in writing

British Library Cataloguing-in-Publication Data
A catalogue record for this book is available from the
British Library

CONTENTS

JOHN HENRY WALSH 1

SECT. 1.—THEIR POSITION IN THE SCALE OF CREATION 7

SECT. 2.—THE NERVOUS SYSTEM 9

SECT. 3.—THE SKELETON 12

SECT. 4.—THE MUSCULAR SYSTEM 29

SECT. 5.—THE ORGANS OF CIRCULATION 33

SECT. 6.—THE ORGANS OF RESPIRATION........... 37

SECT. 7.—THE ORGANS OF NUTRITION AND DEPURATION 46

SECT. 8.—THE ORGANS OF REPRODUCTION 58

SECT. 9.—THE ORGANS OF SENSE 59

SECT. 10.—THE SKIN, AND GENERAL CELLULAR MEMBRANE 60

John Henry Walsh

John Henry Walsh was born on 21 October 1810, in Hackney, London. He is best known as a sports writer, under the pseudonym of 'Stonehenge'. Walsh spent his early education at a nearby private school, before training at the Royal College of Surgeons, passing his examinations in 1831. Soon after Walsh became a fellow of the college, by examination in 1844. He worked in the medical profession for several years, but moved to London in 1852 in order to pursue his love of sports. Walsh had always kept greyhounds and entered them at coursing meetings, becoming especially adept in the management of dogs. Reportedly, few veterinary practitioners could compete with his knowledge of canine diseases. He was also fond of shooting, and, owing to the bursting of his gun, lost a portion of his left hand. In 1853, Walsh, or 'Stonehenge' brought out his first book; *The Greyhound, on the Art of Breeding, Rearing, and Training Greyhounds for public Running, their Diseases and Treatment*. This treatise was based on articles he had written in *Bell's Life*, and, it remains the standard textbook on the subject. Walsh followed up on this books tremendous success with the *Manual of British Rural Sports* (1856), which went through sixteen editions up to 1886 and thereafter encompassed articles on special subjects furnished by other writers. In the same year as the *Manual* was published, Walsh became involved with *The Field* magazine, and accepted the editorship in 1857. He was instrumental in organising the various trials of guns and rifles which *The Field* conducted; most notably a key participator in the controversy as to the merits of breech-loaders and muzzle-loaders, as well as the respective merits of Schultze and black powder. Aside from these endeavours, Walsh was also a founding member of the *All England Lawn Tennis Club*, and was on the committee of the *Kennel Club*. He also played Chess to a good level, and served on the committees of several chess clubs too. Walsh's private life was mired by tragedy however. He was married three times in his life, first in August 1833 to Margaret Stevenson, who died nine months later, secondly to Susan Emily Malden, in 1835, who died eight months later, and thirdly, in 1852 to Louisa Parker, who outlived her husband. Walsh died at 43 Montserrat Road, Putney, Surrey, on 12 February 1888. He is buried at Putney Vale Cemetery at Putney Common.

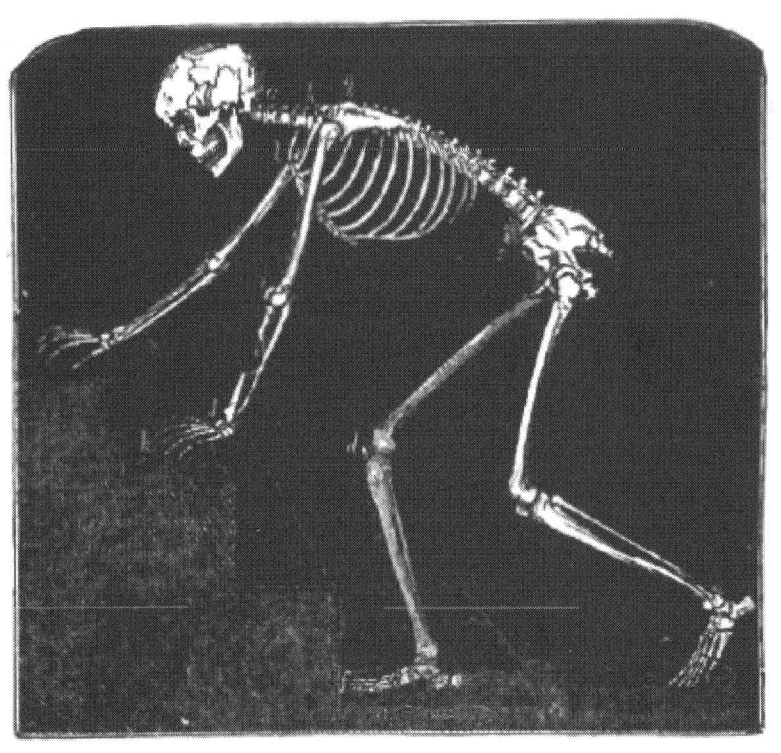

HUMAN SKELETON

BOOK I

COMPARATIVE ANATOMY OF MAN, THE HORSE, AND THE DOG

SECT. 1.—THEIR POSITION IN THE SCALE OF CREATION

MAN himself, together with the horse and the dog, and even the hawk and the decoy-duck, which are the only animals used by him in the capture of the objects of his sport, are all included under the general division *Vertebrata*. These are distinguished by the possession of an articulated skeleton within their bodies, and by a *vertebral column*, containing the most important parts of their nervous system. With the exception of the birds, all the others are included in the class *Mammalia*, so named because they give suck to their young by means of the mammæ. The three species, however, are widely separated in the division, man taking the head of all in a distinct subdivision, and separated from the *Carnivora*, among which the dog is included, by the apes and monkeys. Between the dog, again, and the horse, there intervene the whole of the cetaceous animals and the glires; he horse belonging to the lowest tribe of the mammalia, namely, the *Ungulata*, or those having hoofs. Between these three there will be found to be considerable points of difference in each of the systems of which their frames are composed; all three, however, have a skeleton consisting of the same materials, and containing within its cavities a nervous, a circulatory, a respiratory, a digestive, and a reproductive system. All have the same organs of sense, though differently endowed; and in all the parts of the skeleton are connected together by ligaments forming joints, and moved upon each other by muscles of various forms. The chief differences are—first, in the volume and form of the brain; secondly, in the nature and form of the stomach and intestines; and thirdly, in the form of the organs of locomotion.

SECT. 2.—THE NERVOUS SYSTEM

THE NERVOUS SYSTEM, upon the development of which each animal depends for its position in the scale of creation, is, in the main, the same in the three animals now under consideration. In man, however, it is much more developed in those parts upon which the extent and powers of the mental manifestations and sense of touch are dependent; whilst, in the dog, another part is carried to an exquisite degree of refinement—namely, the nerves in which resides the sense of smell. But in all three there are the same grand portions to be met with, consisting of a mass of highly-complicated nervous matter contained within the skull, called *the brain*, which is the organ of the mind, as well as, in all probability, the seat of the instincts of the animal. Extending from this is a part called the *medulla oblongata*, connecting it with the spinal column, which is chiefly a large bundle of nerves extended between the brain and all the parts of the body below the head, and gradually separating into its component parts as it passes through the bones of the spine. It receives the mandates of the will from the brain, and conveys back to it the state and wants of the various organs of the body.

But, besides these two parts of the nervous system, there are also two others. The first consists of a tract of nervous matter contained within the spinal cord, and intended to supply the organs of respiration, and to keep them in some measure independent of the brain during its sleep, or pressure from accident; and also to effect an action of a very peculiar kind called *reflex*, by which, in certain cases, muscular contractions are produced by a shorter and quicker process than would be afforded by a transmission of the intelligence to the brain itself, and a consequent mandate from it. The second comprises a chain of little brains lying in front of the spine, and within the chest and abdomen, and intended to supply the digestive apparatus and circulating system with nervous influence (whatever that may be), independently of the brain and spinal cord, although these also send their nerves to them. Thus, the most important organs of all have their separate supplies, by which provision is made against accident; and, in case of its occurrence, one part being enabled to do duty for two.

In this way the whole nervous system is divided into—first, the brain; secondly, the medulla oblongata and spinal cord; thirdly, the general nerves of motion and sensation; fourthly, the special nerves of respiration; fifthly, the nerves of the viscera, commonly called the sympathetic system; and, sixthly, the special nerves of the senses derived from the brain itself.

In all the animals named, the nervous system consists of two parts; the grey, in which power is generated, and the white, through which it is transmitted. The grey constitutes the greater part of the exterior of the brain and the interior of the spinal column; whilst the white makes up the interior and central parts of the brain, the exterior of the spinal cord, and the bulk of the nerves of the body.

THE VARIATIONS in these several parts are the following:—In man the brain is much the most voluminous, especially in the anterior part, which is the chief organ of the mind. Here the grey matter is very much convoluted, and thereby rendered more extensive in quantity and in surface, by which his general mental powers are augmented. Next to man in this respect comes the dog, who has sometimes tolerably deep fissures in his brain, and consequently a more extended surface than usual; but in all cases much more so than in the horse, whose brain is, as compared to his whole body, very much less than the dog's, and still more diminished in proportion as compared to that of man. In dogs, however, and especially in those whose powers of smelling are much developed, the anterior lobes, in which the nerves of smelling take their rise, are largely increased in size, and nearly as much so in the horse, who, like all animals dependent upon this sense for their safety in selecting food, has considerable acuteness of smell. In other respects the nervous systems of the three are closely allied, and the description which will serve for the one will also suit the others, except in the minute detail of parts.

SECT. 3.—THE SKELETON

In all three the skeleton consists of the same parts, though the bones composing them vary in number, and to some extent in form. (See skeletons of Man, Dog, and Horse, in which the letters attached to the human skeleton apply also to the corresponding parts in the other two). It is divided into two portions—one forming cavities for containing the vital organs, and protecting them from danger; the other consisting of central supports adapted to the purposes of locomotion, by offering levers to be worked by the various muscles. The bony cavities are—first, the cranium and spinal column; secondly, the thorax or chest attached to the middle of the spine; and, thirdly the pelvis, terminating it. The bony organs of locomotion are the four extremities of the body.

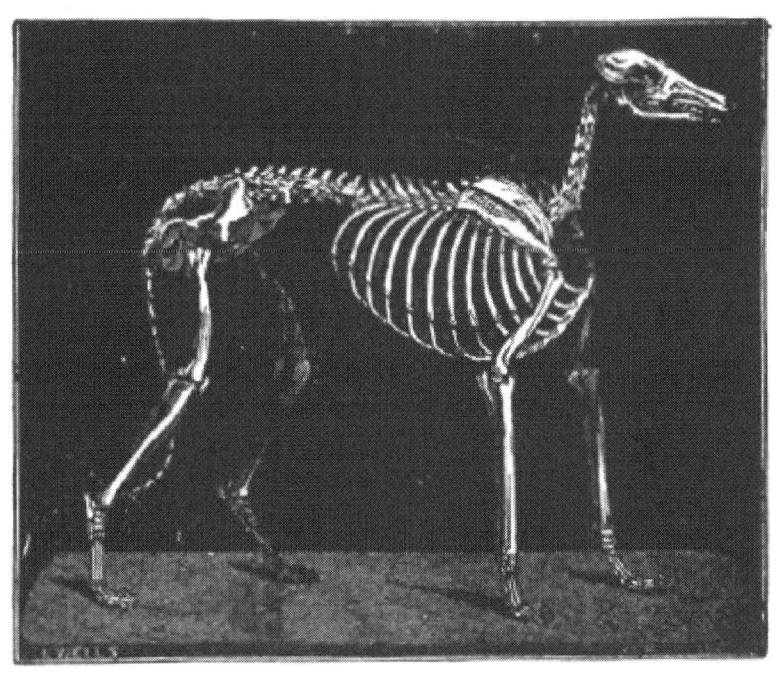

SKELETON OF THE GREYHOUND.

THE CRANIUM OR SKULL, is variously formed in the three species under consideration; but it consists in all three of the same number of bones, eleven of which combine together to form a hollow case for the brain, whilst six of these eleven, together with the upper and lower jawbones, the bones of the nose, and the cheek-bones, constitute the face. In this part they are developed into several cavities, two of which are called the orbits, and contain the eyes; two, close together, form the nostrils; one between the upper and lower jaw-bones, the mouth; and one on each side for the ears, which last part also contains four little delicate bones for communicating the vibrations of the air to the nerve of hearing. In the jaws, also, there are fixed two rows of teeth, the upper and the under, which vary considerably; but in each there are three kinds—viz.: first, the incisors, being more or less cutting nippers, and placed in front; secondly, the canine, pointed, and intended for holding or tearing; and thirdly, the molars, for grinding. The formula, as it is called, for each, is as follows:—

IN MAN.

Incisors, 6/6 Canine, 1/1 : 1/1 Molars, 4/4 : 4/4

IN THE DOG.

Incisors, 6/6 Canine, 1/1 : 1/1 Molars, 6/8 : 6/8

IN THE HORSE.

Incisors, 6/6 Canine, 1/1 : 1/1 Molars, 6/6 : 6/6

The age of man and of the dog can seldom be ascertained by the teeth, but that of the horse may generally be arrived at with tolerable certainty, as follows:—

MARKS OF THE AGE OF THE HORSE AS SHOWN BY THE TEETH.

At one year old, all the milk teeth are come up; the two centre nippers of the lower jaw are partially worn down, the two next very slightly so, and the outside nippers entire.

At two years old, the "mark" is nearly obliterated in the four centre nippers, and those of the outside ones are much reduced in size.

At three years old, the colt has shed the two centre nippers, and has two permanent teeth, on which the "mark" is quite fresh; and the tusks begin to show their future position by a prominence of the gum.

At four years old, the colt has shed the next two milk-teeth, and has four permanent ones, of which the central two are gradually losing their "mark." The tusks now come through, just showing their points.

At five years old, he has all his permanent teeth. The centre nippers are much worn, but still show the "mark." The next are partially worn, while the corner nippers are quite sharp, and with the cavity or "mark" quite untouched by friction. The tusk is much grown, and well raised from the gum.

At six years old, the "mark" in the centre teeth is quite gone, leaving only a yellow oval stain with a black speck in the centre. The next two are also losing their cavity, but the corner teeth are still sharp, and have the cavity unworn to any extent.

At seven years old, the "mark" is gone in all the lower nippers but the corner ones; and

At eight years old, it disappears even there, after which

there is no reliance to be placed upon this sign; the length and *obliquity* of the teeth increase with age in both respects, but these signs depend a good deal upon crib-biting, or other habits, and no great reliance can be placed upon them.

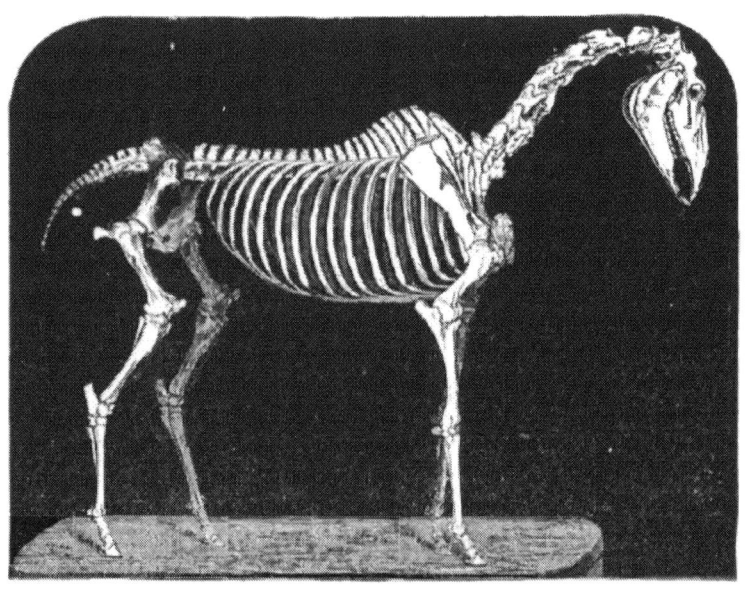

SKELETON OF THE HORSE.

THE SPINAL COLUMN (*a b*) consists in all of a series of bones united together by an elastic material, called the intervertebral substance, and by ligaments also as well as by muscles. Each bone is pierced by a large hole for the lodgment of the spinal cord, and by lesser notches, or holes, for the transmission of the nerves, a pair of which leave the cord opposite each separate bone. Besides the body and the holes (or *foramina*, as they are scientifically called) each vertebra consists of a spinous process, or projection, backwards or upwards, as the case may be; and of another process, or projection on each side, called the lateral process, all of which are intended to secure these bones together, and to give attachment and leverage to the muscles which bend the spine. To the skull the spinal column is attached by a very peculiar universal-hinge-like joint, in such a way that it can be turned in all directions. This in man is very complicated, so as to allow him not only to bend it in all directions, but also to rotate it; whilst in the horse and dog it is strengthened by strong bony projections, so as to support the weight of the head when extended horizontally. The first seven of these bones form the neck, each being more or less lengthened or shortened, according as they are destined to form the long neck of the horse, the medium length of that of the dog, or the short one of man. The next 12 in man, 13 in the dog, and 18 in the horse, have a rib attached to each, or to the intervertebral substance of each, and constitute the vertebræ of the back. Behind or below these are the vertebræ of the loins, which are 5 in man, 6 in the dog, and 7 in the horse; and like those of the neck are free, whilst the last of these lumbar vertebræ is firmly attached in the same way as the others to a corresponding surface of the sacrum, which forms a part of the pelvis, answering to the spinal column, and containing within it a similar canal, which receives the continuation of the spinal cord in the shape of a bundle of nerves, called in anatomy *cauda equina*. Beyond the sacrum, again, are the ossa coccygis, rudimentary in man, but extending to twenty bones in the dog, and in the horse to about fifteen, to form their tails.

THE THORAX, OR CHEST, is formed by the vertebræ of the back and the ribs attached to them, which correspond in number, being in man 12, in the dog 13, and in the horse 18 on each side. Each of them is firmly attached by two joints, one at the end to the intervertebral substance, the other to a lateral process, by means of a tubercle, a short distance from the end. Towards the other extremity the rib becomes flattened, and in its general outline is bent to an irregular segment of a circle, so that the two sides form an arch, more or less of an oval section. Each rib ends by uniting with a piece of cartilage, which in the first seven or eight is directly attached to the sternum, or breast-bone, and in the remainder indirectly through those next to them. The *sternum* consists of a series of spongy bones, comprising 3 in man, and 7 or 8 in the horse and dog, which receive the cartilages, and, with the ribs and the vertebræ of the back, combine to form the chest. In the horse, the front of the sternum projects considerably beyond the first rib, in the dog very little, and in man it has an articulating surface on each side for the attachment of the collar-bone, which is wanting in the horse and dog. In man the greatest diameter, of the chest is from side to side, whilst the reverse is the case in the horse and dog. In each case this cavity contains the lungs and heart and the great vessels, separated from the abdomen by the diaphragm, which is a thin partition of muscle and tendon stretched across so as to form an arch, with the convexity upwards, and a concavity below, against which lie the liver and the stomach—also within the protection of the lower ribs.

THE PELVIS (*b c*) consists of an imperfect circle of strong spongy bone, which is made up of the sacrum and ossa coccygis, or tail bones, above; and of three bones on each side firmly united, called the ilium, the ischium, and the pubes. These together constitute an irregular ring, protecting the bladder and the organs of reproduction, and also giving a firm support to the legs. By a reference to the engravings of the three species, it will be seen that they vary in shape very much. In man the wings of the ilium are much expanded, and serve to support the intestines; or, in the pregnancy of the female, the gravid uterus. In the horse and dog these parts are much less developed, and the whole pelvis is merely a strong bony ring for the articulation of the hind-legs, and for the attachment of muscles; but it will be seen that it is articulated to the sacrum in an oblique direction, so that in coming down from a leap the shock to the nervous system is very much diminished. The tail is merely a prolongation of the ossa coccygis, which in man are contained within the skin, and are simply rudimentary.

The Comparative Anatomy of Man, the Horse, and the Dog

THE HIND-LEGS of the horse and dog and the legs of man are attached to the pelvis in the same way—namely, by means of a ball-and-socket joint; the thigh bone being deeply imbedded in a cup-like cavity of the pelvis, called the *acetabulum*. This is a very strong joint, but it is liable to be dislocated in all three animals; and is in all very difficult of reduction. This leg consists in each of four portions, which in anatomy have received the names of the *femur* (*c d*), *patella* (*d*), *tibia* and *fibula* (*d e*), *tarsus* and *metatarsus* (*e f*); but in common language different names have been given them, which has created considerable confusion.

THE FEMUR—in common language called the *thigh* in man, and the *upper thigh* in the horse and dog—is a long and strong bone, beginning with a smooth ball, called by horsemen the *round bone*, which is deeply let into the cup of the pelvis, and has near it a strong rough process which stands out from it at a considerable angle, and is united to it by a narrow part of the bone called the neck. This process is called the trochanter major, and is the part felt projecting opposite the hip joint; and often called the hip itself, though that name more properly belongs to the crest or ridge of the ilium. Towards the lower end the thighbone enlarges and forms a smooth surface, covered with cartilage and extending to nearly three-fourths of a circle from before backwards. This smooth surface is attached by strong ligaments to the tibia below, and has playing upon it in front a bone called the patella in anatomy, or in common language the *knee-cap* in man, and the *stifle-bone* in the horse and dog. The joint itself is the *knee* in man, and the *stifle* in ordinary equine and canine nomenclature; but. being more or less concealed in them by the flank and large muscles of the thigh, it is overlooked by superficial observers. This joint in all three is liable to accidents, or to inflammations of a serious character, and is frequently the seat of lameness.

THE TIBIA—called in man the *leg-bone*, and in the horse and dog the *lower thigh bone*—extends from the stifle joint to the hock in the latter two animals, and from the knee to the ankle in man, It is supported by a smaller bone on the outside (the fibula), which is lost sight of in common language, and has received no distinctive appellation. In man this bone forms a part of the ankle-joint; but in the dog and horse, the hock joint (which corresponds to the ankle of man) is composed of the tibia alone, as regards its upper boundary, whilst below, in all cases, it is made up by the upper bone of the tarsus—namely, the astragalus.

THE TARSUS AND METATARSUS vary more in these three species than any other parts of the skeleton, except the corresponding divisions of the other extremity. In man and in the dog the tarsus consists of seven bones, but in the horse of six only. In all, however, the tibia is articulated with the tarsus at about one-half of the length from the hind end, and by a cartilaginous surface, composed of three sides; there is also in each a projecting bone (the *os calcis*), which affords leverage to the strong muscles of the tibia and femur, ending in a tendon, which is called the tendo-Achillis. These bones are united together into a strong whole by ligaments and intervening cartilage, which take off the jar that would otherwise be communicated to the body when the springs and falls are sustained which all these animals are subject to. Below the tarsus are the metatarsal bones—five in man, four in the dog, and limited to one only in the horse, the *cannon*, though with a rudimentary bone on each side, called the *splent bone*. In all of these animals they are tipped by three phalanges to each metatarsal bone, except in man, who has only two to the great toe. In the horse the first phalanx is called the *larger pastern*, the second the *smaller pastern*, and the third the *coffin bone:* whilst the sesamoid bone behind it, which is also found in man and the dog, receives the name of the *navicular bone;* and all are surmounted by horny matter constituting the nails of man and the dog, and the hoofs of the horse. There is, however, this grand difference between the three—man walks upon the whole length of the tarsus, metatarsus, and phalanges, or upon the sole of the foot (*planta*), and is hence called *plantigrade;* but the dog and horse walk upon the tips of their fingers only, and are called *digitigrade* for that reason— the former walking upon all his fingers, whilst the latter walks upon one only, the remainder being lost in the splent bones, which do not reach the length of the fingers at all. Both carry their hocks (corresponding with our heels) some distance from the ground, whilst ours is the first part to touch it in the walk; and it is only in the run upon the toes that it is carried clear of the ground.

All these several points of resemblance or difference will be rendered clearer by comparing the skeleton of man, purposely placed in a stooping position, with those of the dog and horse. A side view of each is given in a corresponding attitude; and thus it may be seen how our knee is the same joint with their stifles; how our heel is their hock; and in what way our foot corresponds with their pasterns, and our metatarsal bones with the *cannon bone* of the horse; also, how our nails are analogous to the hoofs of the horse, which grow in the same way, or nearly so, and are as easily separated by inflammation, or other disease.

THE UPPER EXTREMITY of man corresponds with the fore-leg of his chief ministers, the dog and horse, but differs still more than is the case with the other extremity, which is chiefly used by man in progressing, though in a different position to that of the dog and horse, he being a biped. But with the limb we are now considering, a hundred different actions are to be performed—ropes are to be pulled down or up, or straight towards the body; large and small substances are to be grasped in the arms; hammers are to be wielded with terrific force, or with all the delicacy necessary for riveting the fine mechanism of a watch; besides the multifarious movements of a similar character. But in addition to all these motions, requiring the whole limb, there are others depending upon the fore-arm alone, in which man shows his superiority to the dog and horse. If the former of these has a wound in the sole of his foot, he is obliged to lie down and forcibly push it sideways against the ground, while he bends the foot, in order that he may get at it with his tongue. Man, on the other hand, can readily turn his palm upwards, and at once detect the mischief, if any there be. In other words, *man can pronate and supinate his hand*, a gift of immeasurable importance to him, though one which he shares with all the higher genera of the monkey tribe. By this power he can turn any object about as he fashions it to his purpose, and can with the greatest ease do that which the otherwise intelligent dog is incapable of effecting. Hence we find that throughout the whole extremity, although the same bones are made subsidiary to this new purpose, yet they are widely different in their joints, and also vary in general form. Nevertheless, all have a shoulder-blade, a humerus, a radius and ulna, and a carpus and a metacarpus. Man, also, has a collar-bone, by which the shoulder-blade is attached to the breast-bone, and is thus rendered more completely a fixed point for the various operations, often antagonistic to each other, which his wants demand.

THE SHOULDER-BLADE (*g h*) is very similar in all three skeletons in its general form, though varying considerably in position and in the detail of its parts. In each case it is a triangular flat bone, with a ridge dividing its external surface into two parts. In all there is a shallow cup which receives the head of the humerus, and forms with it the *shoulder joint* of man, and the *point of the shoulder* of the horse and dog. Protecting this joint in man, and partially so in the dog, are two projecting points of bone, the *acromion* and *coracoid processes*, to which the outer extremity of the COLLARBONE (*h l*) is firmly united by strong ligaments, the other end being still more securely confined to the breast-bone by a thick intervening cartilage and additional ligaments. Here there is a strong point of dissimilarity, the dog and horse neither of them possessing a collar-bone; but it is not confined to man, since many of the lower animals also possess collar-bones; as, for instance, the hare, rabbit, and rat—and, in fact, all the division Rodentia; most of which, however, require and possess, like him, the power of grasping their food, and can pronate and supinate their fore-arms to a degree almost equal to that with which he is endowed. The shoulder-blade in man does not lie so flat on his sides as in the dog and horse, its outer aspect looking nearly in the same direction as his spine; whilst in the other two it looks directly outwards, or very nearly so, the free margins approaching one another more than the joints.

THE HUMERUS (*h i*) is very similar in its general form in all three, presenting a rounded articular surface at the upper end, a long cylindrical middle, and an oblong smooth ridge covered with cartilage at the other extremity, which forms part of a hinge-like joint, the remainder being made up by the ulna and radius. This bone in man is called *the arm*, or the *upper arm;* and in the horse and dog the *true arm*, being in them concealed within the body by the muscles and skin with which it is clothed. In all three the joint bounding it below is called the *elbow-joint*.

THE ULNA AND RADIUS (*i j*) are articulated to the humerus, so as to form a simple hinge in the horse and dog, as well as in man; but in addition there is another power given to man, to which I have already alluded, and which is carried out by a very simple yet effective contrivance. In him the ulna forms the chief part of the elbow-joint, whilst the radius enters into that of the wrist, and each has a liberty of rotating in its attachment at the opposite end. Thus, the two may be compared to one bone of somewhat greater length, and joined to the elbow and wrist in the usual way, but afterwards divided obliquely from one end to the other in such a way as to leave one joint entire for the wrist, and the other for the elbow. If this were done by a carpenter, and the bones rounded off and attached together by a circle of leather at each end, it would be found that there would be a degree of liberty similar to that which we enjoy, but not quite to so great an extent, which is afforded by the two bones arching out from one another in the middle, and thus enabling the movement to be still more complete. The ulna is the bone chiefly entering into the composition of the elbow-joint; and it, like the hock and ankle, has a process projecting backwards, for the purpose of giving leverage to its muscles, which is the *olecranon* in anatomy, or the *point of the elbow* in common language, in all three animals. The radius in the dog extends to the *carpus*, but in the horse it does not reach so far; together they form the *fore-arm* in man, and the *true arm* in the horse and dog.

THE CARPUS AND METACARPUS (*j k*).—The former consists of eight bones in man, and of seven in the horse and dog; and in this joint there is very little difference between them. In all there are strong ligaments connecting the bones together, so as to form one strong whole, with a projecting hooklike process standing back, under cover of which the flexor tendons pass behind the wrist, and are securely bound in their places. In man the lower row of bones is articulated with the five *metacarpal bones*, which spread to form the palm of the hand. In the dog there are four and in the horse one, which, like the metatarsal bone of the hind-leg, is called the *cannon bone*, and is also supported by two rudimentary metatarsals and *splent bones* of the fore-leg.

THE HAND OF MAN is a complex mechanism, composed of the five metacarpal bones, four of which each carry three phalanges to form the fingers, and the fifth two only for the thumb. These are simple enough in their bony mechanism, but when clothed with their numerous muscles, and furnished with the net-work of vessels and nerves which the sense of touch requires, it is indeed a wonderful and exquisitely delicate machine—capable alike of picking up the most minute speck of sand, or of wielding the ponderous hammer of the smith. In the horse and dog the phalanges are almost precisely similar to those of the hind extremity.

SECT. 4.—THE MUSCULAR SYSTEM

THE MUSCLES are the powers which chiefly effect the various movements, either of one part of the body upon another, or of it as a whole upon the surface of the earth. These movements are sometimes produced by the simple expansion and contraction of hollow muscles, as in the heart, stomach, &c.; or by means of the attachment of the two ends of a muscle to two separate bones with an intervening joint. The description of the precise mode by which muscles contract is too deep and abstruse a part of physiological science for a book intended for the sportsman; but it may simply be stated as a fact, that all muscles have the power of contraction, either at the mandate of the will, or at the command of some other power inherent in particular parts of the nervous system. The former set of muscles are called the *voluntary* muscles, and are those by which we walk, talk, sing, &c.; whilst the latter are those which contract upon the food in the stomach and intestines, or upon the blood in the heart, &c., without our knowledge and consent, and are hence called *involuntary*: a third set, again, are usually involuntary, but sometimes voluntary, as the muscles of respiration and of the bladder and rectum. But besides this division of muscles into voluntary, involuntary, and mixed, there is another which includes nearly the same sets of muscles in its two sections—the first of which clothes the skeleton, and moves its various parts upon one another; whilst the second incloses the hollow viscera, and contracts upon them, but has no bony attachments. The first of these includes the voluntary muscles, and those mixed muscles which are concerned in respiration and in closing the various orifices; whilst the second comprehends the involuntary muscles, and those mixed ones which contract upon the bladder and rectum.

THE MUSCLES WHICH ACT UPON THE SKELETON are very similar in general form and action in man, the dog, and the horse; and, as is the case with the skeleton, the same names have been adopted into comparative anatomy which were originally given to the muscles of man. There are, however, numerous points of difference, the complicated hand and fore-arm of man requiring many more muscles than the corresponding parts in the dog and horse. In all cases, however, they are adapted by their contraction to bring two different bones together, either in their whole length, as in the case of the ribs, or at one extremity only of each, as in the long bones. In the ribs the movements are made by two sets of fibres crossing one another, so that they do not act directly from the edge of one to that of the next, but obliquely, by which they are enabled to bring the two edges much nearer together than would be the case if they acted in a straight direction. It is a rule in all cases that muscles act with power proportioned to their size, but with an extent in accordance with their length. Hence, a short but broad and thick muscle is exceedingly strong, but cannot effect such extensive movements as another which is longer but thinner. Sometimes, again, as around joints, space is an object, and here the muscular fibre is replaced by tendon, which is a firm band or cord of white and comparatively insensible fibrous matter, to which the contractile muscular fibres are intimately connected, and through which they act. Thus, this department of the muscular system is made up—first, of large masses of muscles attached directly to bone at each end, or with scarcely any tendinous insertion, as those of the shlouder and buttock; secondly, of muscles consisting of a middle muscular part called *the belly*, and of one or more tendinous cords, as in the muscles of the fore-arm, &c.; and thirdly, of a thin sheet of muscle ending in a still thinner sheet of strong tendon, as in those of the abdomen. These muscles are bound down in their places by *fascia*, a thin but strong membrane; and when their tendons pass behind joints they are confined in their proper grooves by still firmer and stronger fibrous tissue, forming a complete sheath for them, and called a *theca*. These as well as the joints are lubricated by a mucilaginous oil, called *synovia;* and, in many cases, beneath muscles which pass over bones, there is a bag of the same lubricating fluid, called a *bursa mucosa*. In all the limbs the muscles are arranged in two groups, one which bends the joints, and the other to extend them; but very often when a long muscle passes over two joints, it is a flexor of one and an extensor of the other.

THE HOLLOW MUSCLES vary in thickness and in complexity of structure, from the heart, with its cavities and its numerous valves, to the simple, thin, and circular fibres of the intestines.

The heart will be described under the Organs of Circulation, and the muscles of the stomach and bowels under the Digestive Organs.

SECT. 5.—THE ORGANS OF CIRCULATION

THE HEART AND BLOOD VESSELS are intended to circulate the blood throughout the whole body, including the lungs; and in the three species we are now examining they are nearly identical, the only difference being such as to allow of the upright position of man. The whole body, being built up from the blood, must be liberally supplied with it, in proportion to the duties of the several organs; this is effected by means of a series of tubes beginning with one trunk, dividing and subdividing like the branches of a tree, and spreading over the body, the whole inside and outside of which are furnished from this source with arterial blood, as the material by which they are kept in order and growth, and from which the various organs secrete or excrete the bile, the urine, perspiration, saliva, &c. These vessels are called the arteries, and they end in a set of minute tubes, called the *capillaries*, from their fineness, which is compared to that of a hair (*capillus*). The capillaries, again, are connected with the extreme branches of another set of tubes, still more numerous than the arteries, and of greater aggregate bulk, which receive the blood through the capillaries from the arteries, and finally end in two veins—the superior and inferior *venæ cavæ*, which force the blood back again into the heart. They are furnished with valves at regular distances, wherever the flow is at all impeded by muscular action or position, as in the legs, arms, &c. This is the mode by which the blood is circulated throughout the body, being propelled by the contractile power of the heart, aided by that of the arteries through their whole course, and also through the capillaries and veins, till it returns back to the heart.

But the blood does not at once proceed on its round again. A cleansing process must be effected; for in its course it has changed its appearance and its properties, going out scarlet and coming back purple, and having lost oxygen and absorbed carbon—in fact, having been converted from arterial to venous blood, and being no longer fitted for the various duties which the blood is required to perform. It is no doubt a living fluid, and endowed with properties of which we cannot fathom the nature; but from experiment we have arrived at the conclusion that the above changes are produced, and that it requires the contact with atmospheric air, with the intervention only of a very thin membrane, in order to restore to it its oxygen, and to remove its carbon. It is also found by experiment, that air after it is expired contains more carbon than before, in the shape of carbonic acid gas, and has lost part of its free oxygen; hence the conclusion is arrived at that the blood has effected this exchange in its passage through the lungs. This is somewhat similar to what goes on in our stoves, where oxygen and carbon combine to form carbonic acid gas;

and in both cases there is an evolution of heat. The blood, therefore, must pass through the lungs for this purpose; and it is forced into them by a separate artery (the pulmonary), and returned from them by the pulmonary veins; the arteries in this case carrying venous blood, and the veins bringing back arterial blood to the heart. Thus, there are two distinct circulations going on in our bodies—one driving the blood through all parts, and bringing it back to the heart; the other, forcing this same current through the lungs, and back again to the same heart, but to a different cavity.

THE HEART itself may be said to be composed of two forcing-pumps tied together, each of which consists of a thin receiving cavity (the auricle), and of a strong propelling cavity (the ventricle), with valves between. These are called respectively the right and left sides of the heart. The right auricle, in this way, receives the venous blood from the whole body, and forces it into the right ventricle, out of which it is prevented from returning into the auricle by a valve. The ventricle, contracting, forces the blood into the lungs, through the pulmonary arteries, and back through the pulmonary veins into the left auricle; this again passes it into the left ventricle, which, being also guarded by a valve, propels it through the aorta to all parts of the body, and so completes this beautiful circle.

Besides these blood-vessels, there is also a set of *absorbent vessels*, of whose powers we know very little, except that they take up and convey into the large veins a part of the fluids and solids of the body; but how far they are assisted by the veins, or in what way the work is divided between them, has never been fully ascertained. They are very fine, colourless, and transparent tubes, arising in all parts of the body, and passing through certain organs called *absorbent glands*, finally emptying themselves in the large veins near the heart.

THE PULSE.—The heart propels the blood with such force through the arteries, that in the principal one of the neck of the horse, if a tube is attached to it, a column is raised ten feet high, and maintained at that average level. The power and frequency of the contractions varies much, from 100 beats a minute in the small dog to 40 per minute in the horse. In these contractions the arteries, as they receive the blood, elongate and expand, and then contract upon their contents, so as to make what was at first an intermittent action resolve itself into a continuous one as the blood reaches the small vessels. Hence the flow from a large artery is by jets, and from small ones continuous. This alternate action and reaction of the heart upon the artery, and of the artery upon the blood, constitutes what is called *the pulse*, which may be felt in the situation of any large artery, but is generally examined in man at the wrist, in the dog under the arm, and in the horse under the lower jaw, opposite the middle grinders.

SECT. 6.—THE ORGANS OF RESPIRATION

In the last section I have briefly alluded to the process which is effected in the organs of respiration, by which the blood is renovated, and animal heat is evolved. The heart has been shown to throw its blood through the lungs, and it must now be explained that these consist of a spongy texture, made up of fine air-cells, communicating with each other, and with small air-tubes (*bronchi*), which finally unite by means of a single bronchus on each side of the *trachea*, or *windpipe*. This, again, passes up the neck, and at the root of the tongue it is guarded by a complex mechanism, consisting of several cartilages, ligaments, and muscles, by which foreign bodies are prevented entering and producing irritation; and where, also, the various sounds are effected which in man constitute his language, and in dogs and horses, barking, growling, neighing, &c. This is called the *larynx*. Into the cells of this spongy texture the air is admitted, and from them it is expelled by the act of breathing; and while there it is separated from the blood circulating over their walls by the thin membraneous lining of the cells, and by the coats of the capillaries themselves. The substance of the lungs themselves is made up of a lining membrane, which extends over the whole inner surface of the cells and air-tubes, and which secretes the mucus that keeps them moist, and is continuous with the mucous membrane of the mouth at the top of the larynx.

The lungs are divided into two large sections, one on each side of the body, which again are subdivided into lobes; but the grand division is into the two lungs; and they each lie within their respective sides of the chest; and they, as well as the internal surface of the ribs, are, as it were, varnished by a thin membrane, called the *pleura*. This membrane is carried from one to the other in such a way that it forms a large shut sac, the outside of which is applied, on the one hand, to the inside of the ribs; on another, to the outside of the lungs; and on a third, to the upper surface of the diaphragm, which forms the lower boundary of the thorax. This cavity usually contains a very small, and almost inappreciable quantity of serum, secreted in the inside, and enabling the various lobes of the lungs to glide smoothly against the walls of the chest. Between these two membranes, the serous on the outside and the mucous on the inside, there is a small quantity of fine cellular membrane, in which lie the blood vessels and nerves, and which is called the *parenchyma*, or substance, of the lungs in anatomy. Each of these tissues is the seat of a separate inflammation, and their nature and functions should be known in order to treat them properly.

But, though I have shown how the blood is propelled through the lungs, and that these are capable of admitting air to it for the purpose of renewing its requisite properties, there remains to be described the mechanism by which this air is admitted and renewed—and this in proportion to the impurity of the blood, whether healthy, the effect of exercise, or unhealthy, as in disease. In order to understand this mechanism, the chamber in which the lungs lie must be examined, when it will be found to consist of an irregular cone with the narrow part towards the neck of the animal. The sides of this cone are composed of a series of hoops, which do not form segments of circles, but are more or less angular in their curves, and are attached obliquely to the bones of the spine, which are fixed points, so that as they are raised they increase the diameter greatly; but in man and in the horse and dog in a very different mode. In man they may be considered as a series of hoops which rise and fall like the hood of a carriage, the breast-bone merely connecting the two sets of ribs, and rising together with them. In him. therefore, the diameter is increased almost entirely from behind forwards, and not to any great extent from side to side. In the dog and horse, on the contrary, the spine and breast-bone are both of them fixed points, and the ribs on each side are raised independently of each other, increasing the transverse, but not the perpendicular diameter. The reason for this difference is, that these animals are both suspended from their ribs to their shoulder-blades; and if they were continually altering the position of their breast-bones, as regards their spines, they must also raise and lower their bodies, which would be a great and unnecessary expenditure of muscular force; whilst by dilating their chests only laterally, the attachments of the great suspensory muscle are always at the same distance from each other; and whether the lungs are dilated or contracted, the body is at the same distance from the ground. Place a man panting for breath flat upon his breast, and observe how his body rises and falls with each inspiration and expiration, and he will tell you at the same time how much more laborious his breathing is; just so would it be with those animals whose bodies are required to be supported upon stable points, however elastic may be the connecting medium, and not upon a movable frame, which in the horse, if his chest moved like that of man, would rise two or three inches with every inspiration. For this reason it is that many flat-sided horses and dogs are good-winded, because, though their chests are not naturally capacious, yet from their capability of increasing the cavity rapidly, they can change the volume of air more completely than a rounder and larger-barrelled animal, whose ribs are not so movable. Every one has heard the schoolboy's riddle, which demands—"How is it possible to arrange a hundred sheep-hurdles so that two more shall enable the fold to contain double the number of sheep?" The answer being, by placing them in two straight lines, leaving only a narrow space of the width of a hurdle between them; the volume is doubled by a slight increase of width. So it is with a narrow chest, if only the ribs are set on with a good curve, and the muscles have power to bear them.

Besides this increase of the capacity of the chest by means of the ribs, there is another and most important aid in the diaphragm, a muscular and tendinous division, of an arched form, which separates the chest from the abdomen, lying completely across with its convexity towards the lungs. This convexity is capable of being diminished to a plane surface, by its contraction; and in the living state, especially during its powerful action when strong exercise is going on, there is reason to believe that it becomes nearly or quite plane, whilst it is afterwards rendered convex again by means of the abdominal muscles, which force the liver and stomach into its concave surface, and thus push it against the lungs themselves, and expel their air.

In this way, the muscles attached to the ribs increasing the transverse diameter, and the diaphragm enlarging the cavity towards the abdomen, the air is strongly drawn through the trachea into the interior of the lungs, and expelled again by the muscles which lower the ribs, and by the abdominal muscles pushing up the liver and stomach, as well as by the natural elasticity of the lungs themselves, and of the walls of the chest. In ordinary respiration, the inspirations are chiefly carried on by the diaphragm; but in violent struggles, which demand all the air that can be forced in, the shoulder-blades, arms, neck, and head all become fixed, because they have muscles attached to them, and to the ribs also, which in the usual way are employed in moving these various organs, but which now become auxiliary to respiration by acting upon the ribs from these several parts as fixed points. Hence, the runner keeps his arms well up and fixed, and his head and neck stiff, because in this way instinct teaches him that his ribs are more forcibly raised than they would be with lowered shoulders, flaccid arms, and drooping chin. The horse also extends his neck, and by so much helps to raise his ribs on each side; but he does not set his shoulder-blades, for two reasons—first, because it would interfere with his progress in the gallop; and secondly, because the muscles which run from the shoulder-blade to the ribs are not auxiliary muscles of respiration, for they have no power to act upon the ribs in the way in which only their action would be serviceable—that is, towards the apex of the chest, which is also the root of the neck, where the really useful auxiliaries are attached.

THE CHEMICAL ACTION of respiration is more mysterious than the mechanical, for though much has been discovered by Liebig and others, there is still a great deal which is incomprehensible. It will, in the first place, be necessary to explain that the atmospheric air is made up of 21 parts of oxygen to 79 of nitrogen, which is the condition in which it enters the lungs, whilst on its reappearance it has sustained the following changes—first, it has lost oxygen; secondly, it has received carbon in the form of carbonic acid; thirdly, it has suffered a change in the quantity of nitrogen, varying with the condition of the animal. These changes are intimately connected with the effect upon the blood, which is found at the same time to have gained what the air has lost, and to have given out exactly what the air has gained; and thus it is conclusively ascertained that the air is inspired for this express purpose. The absorbed oxygen is supposed by Liebig to enter then and there into combination with the carbon, which process he describes as exactly similar to ordinary combustion; but, from other experiments, there is strong reason to believe that the oxygen is absorbed into the blood, and that its union with the carbon takes place in all the parts of the body; the carbonic acid being there generated and contained in the veins until they reach the lungs and skin, where it is given out; so that the combustion is a general one, and animal heat is thus produced in the extremities, independently of the warm blood sent them from the heart. But besides this oxygen absorbed for this specific purpose, a still further quantity is absorbed for the purpose of uniting with the sulphur and phosphorus contained in the body, by which they are enabled to combine with other elements, and so produce the phosphates and sulphates.

The carbon which is exhaled from the lungs and skin is of an enormous amount, varying with the exercise taken, and with the temperature of the surrounding air—a great quantity of the former and a low degree of the latter both increasing the exhalation of carbon. By actual experiment it has been found, that a person who, in a state of rest and fasting, excreted 145 grains per hour, after a meal and a walk excreted 190 in the same time. During sleep the same person only excreted 100 grains. It is supposed that an adult male who takes strong exercise will excrete about 10 or 11 oz. per 24 hours; and that those who take little will not lose more than 7 or 8 ounces. Assuming 10 oz. as the average, its union with oxygen to form carbonic acid gas will produce 21 cubic feet of that noxious element. So that a man lying in a confined space of 7 feet long by 3 feet wide, will, in the course of 24 hours, discharge from his person enough carbonic acid gas to fill this space 1 foot high; and as carbonic acid is much heavier, and very slowly mixes with the general atmosphere, he would, if lying perfectly flat, destroy his life by suffocation, unless there happened to be some leakage under doors and similar apertures. This fact should be borne in mind in the construction of stables, where the area for each horse is seldom more than 100 superficial feet; and, as the weight of his body is more than five times greater than that of man, it will be manifest that he will also give off during the same time enough carbonic acid gas to fill his stall or box to the same height; and it is only the presence of the crevice under the doors, *and very often of open drains untrapped*, which saves him from the injurious effects of this gas.

The examination of the nitrogen which is given off or absorbed is not of so much importance to our present subject, especially as little is known of its effects; but it is found that animals well fed and in health increase the nitrogen already existing in the air, whilst those which are badly fed absorb it, and consequently diminish its amount in the air; thus, in hibernating animals, nitrogen and oxygen are actually absorbed to a greater extent than they exhale carbon; and hence they do not lose weight during the period of their long sleep.

The following table shows the difference of the proportions of these elements in the two states of the blood:—

	Arterial Blood.	Venous Blood.
Carbonic acid	62·3	71·6
Oxygen	23·2	15·3
Nitrogen	14·5	13·1
Total	100	100

Thus, it would appear that the quantity of nitrogen is very nearly the same in both conditions of the blood; whilst about one-third of the free oxygen of the arterial blood disappears during its circulation and passage into the veins, and is replaced by an equivalent amount of carbonic acid. The converse of this takes place in the capillary vessels of the pulmonary vessels, where this same amount of carbonic acid is set free and replaced by oxygen.

SECT. 7.—THE ORGANS OF NUTRITION AND DEPURATION

In all animals there is a constant necessity for the repair of the waste going on in the various processes, such as muscular contraction, respiration, &c. This repair must be accomplished by means of food; and it is further necessary that digestion shall prepare this food previously to its being converted into that generally useful fluid, the blood, from which all the materials of the body are built.

THE BLOOD, as seen by the microscope in the living vessels, is composed of two parts—one transparent, thin, and nearly colourless, called *liquor sanguinis;* the other consisting of *corpuscles*, some of which are red, and others colourless, but all more or less disk-shaped. When blood is drawn from the body, there is a different separation, into *clot* and *serum*. The former is composed of a network of *fibrine*, in which the corpuscles are entangled, while the latter is identical with the liquor sanguinis, but deprived of its fibrine. The serum also contains a quantity of *albumen*, which coagulates by heat; and likewise earthy salts, which remain after it is evaporated and exposed to a high temperature. This gives us the four following components of the blood, differently arranged in the living vessels, and when deprived of their protection:—

	BLOOD IN THE LIVING VESSELS
	consists of
Fibrine, Albumen, Salts,	{ Forming with water the liquor sanguinis, in which are suspended the corpuscles.

	BLOOD, WHEN DRAWN AND COAGULATED,
	consists of
Fibrine and Corpuscles,	{ Forming the clot, with small quantity of water.
Albumen and Salts,	{ Forming with a larger proportion of water the serum and remaining fluid.

THE USE of these various materials is as follows:—

1.—THE FIBRINE is the material which is most thoroughly elaborated, and ready for supplying the muscles and other solid tissues with new matter, in lieu of their worn-out atoms. It is, therefore, continually being employed for these purposes, and fresh supplies afforded, partly by absorption directly from the digested food and partly from the conversion of albumen into fibrine in the blood-vessels themselves, which is constantly going on in the circulation of the blood.

2.—THE ALBUMEN is the next in point of importance, being also the most abundant, and not only keeping up by its conversion the requisite quantity of fibrine, but also directly supplying many of the secretions and formations, as the scarf-skin, nails, horns, and a great part of the skin itself, also the soft parts of the bones, and, in fact, all the gelatinous tissues, as well as, in all probability, the corpuscles themselves.

3.—THE CORPUSCLES are chiefly useful in carrying on the process of respiration, and in stimulating the contractions of the muscular tissues; but the presence of the red corpuscles is no doubt necessary to the health and well-being of all the warm-blooded vertebrated animals.

4.—THE SALINE MATTER is partly required in order to prevent decomposition, and, in part, to supply the mineral materials necessary for the formation of bone, in which lime and phosphorus are chiefly concerned; and also for the secretion of some of the fluids which are necessary for the purposes of digestion—as the bile, saliva, pancreatic fluid, &c.

5.—THE WATER is, as in all other cases, the means of making fluid the otherwise solid materials.

THE SUPPLY OF FRESH BLOOD is kept up by the *digestion* and *assimilation* of food admitted into the stomach for that purpose; hence it would appear that for a healthy individual, food which contains all the essential elements of blood, in the proportions adapted to his particular state, is the best calculated to support the waste of the system. Thus, supposing an animal is largely consuming his muscular apparatus by long-continued and violent exercise, then food which contains in large proportions the elements necessary for the repair of muscular tissue, will be best adapted for his state. Or in case of an animal exposed to severe cold, his condition will be most improved by supplying him with food in which carbon is a principal ingredient, because we know that this elementary substance is the one which is engaged in producing animal heat. The first and most important process, therefore, in nutrition is the procuration of proper food.

DIGESTION is the next step in the circle of needful processes, and by this is understood the prehension, deglutition, maceration, and chemical conversion of the food into what is called *chyme*—a pulpy fluid, which is ready to be changed into *chyle*, and at once absorbed into the blood by the vessels specially appointed for that purpose. Now, the seizing, masticating, swallowing, and maceration in the stomach, of the articles of food, is managed somewhat differently in the three species under consideration; man employing various agents, such as fire, water, mechanical trituration, &c., to assist him; and the dog using his teeth and paws, to gnaw his bones and tear the flesh into shreds before he swallows it. The horse, on the other hand, crops the grass with his incisors, or gathers up the corn with his lips, and grinds the latter well into a pulpy mash before he swallows it. In these several ways, and by the aid of the saliva, the food is masticated and swallowed by them all, and reaches the stomach more or less prepared for the dissolving power which that organ possesses in such a remarkable degree.

In man and the dog the stomach is capable of holding a very considerable meal, being in all probability intended by nature for long fasts and occasional replenishments only—not perhaps exceeding one meal a day, as is the usual custom with savage tribes, who indeed gorge themselves, and then fast with an endurance which civilized nations cannot possibly imitate. The same change has taken place in the dog's stomach by civilization, and he now is rarely suffered to pass twenty-four hours without two or three meals; when in his natural state there can be no doubt he would scarcely average three or four full meals a week. The horse, on the other hand, when in his native plains, is perpetually feeding in small portions at a time; and he then, as now, requires small and regular supplies of food at short intervals, to keep him in a state of full health. By many this is supposed to be in order to enable him to gallop without injury; but it is rather that he may *always* be prepared for flight, because, unlike the carnivorous animals, he cannot choose his time, but must save himself by the use of his heels, whether after a full meal or a light one. The dog, on the other hand, can gorge himself and wait till he is again hungry before he exerts his powers; and he may consequently be furnished with a capacious stomach without risk. Man, also, has the same choice, and, like the dog, he fills himself, and then sleeps till his stomach warns him that he must replenish it by the chase.

The stomach consists, in all three, of an oval sac, with an orifice at one end by which it receives its food, and another at the other end, through which it passes it out into the small intestines as soon as it is fit for the manufacture of *chyle*. It has an outside covering, smooth and lubricated with serous fluid, which suffers it to assume the various forms which its change from a state of emptiness to one of repletion demands. Next to this serous coat is a muscular one, which serves to contract the various parts, and so move the food from one to the other; and lining this, again, is the mucous surface, studded with small glands, by which the *gastric juice*, the main agent of digestion, is produced, and also sufficient mucus to protect the walls of the stomach from its powers, or from any deleterious article admitted into it by mistake. This juice is a very powerful solvent, and is made up of various acids and other powerful agents, by which even bones themselves are dissolved in the stomach of the dog, and also sometimes in that of man. It is not present in the empty stomach, but is poured out rapidly as soon as food is introduced, and soon changes it into the pulpy substance which I have already said is called chyme. This is semi-fluid, and with a slight acid taste, sometimes creamy in appearance when the food is oily, or more like gruel when farinaceous. Part of this is at once absorbed through the walls of the stomach itself, and conveyed direct into the blood; the remainder passes on by the agency of the muscular fibres into the *duodenum*, or first small intestine, where it is mixed with the *bile* and with the *pancreatic juice*, and becomes converted into a still more pulpy and milky fluid, the *chyle*, which is passed on into the remainder of the small intestines, the *jejunum* and *ilium*, and there is taken up by the chyliferous absorbents, called lacteals, and conveyed into the large vein near the heart by a particular absorbent tube, called the *thoracic duct*. The remainder, which is not absorbed, is passed on by the muscular contractions of the bowels, called *peristaltic*, to the larger intestines; and there becoming still further relieved of its watery particles, and also receiving the addition of some worn-out materials poured in from the blood-vessels surrounding their coats, it finally assumes the appearance of *fæces*, and is discharged *per anum*.

THE BILE AND PANCREATIC FLUID are both concerned in the preparation of the chyle, to which duties they are specially appointed; but over and above this it appears that the bile is useful in depurating the blood, and removing from it certain noxious elements, which, if retained, would become highly injurious. The pancreatic fluid is only secreted during digestion, but the bile is poured out at all times; and, if not secreted because of any torpid condition of the liver, the blood becomes overloaded with noxious particles, headache follows, and finally, fever and even fatal injury. Bile is a kind of soap, and appears to act specially in converting sugar into albumen and the fatty compounds necessary for the support of life. The pancreatic fluid, on the other hand, seems to render the fat taken as food fit for absorption, which it is not in its raw state. But not only is the liver useful by supplying bile, but it also directly purifies the blood as it passes through it in the return from the intestines to the heart; and besides this, it seems to exert a powerful influence in *assimilating* the new material to the condition which it must attain as a part of the blood. Here also fibrine is largely formed from albumen, and fat from sugar.

THE KIDNEYS AND SKIN still further purify the blood, and remove the watery particles which are introduced into it as a solvent for the various solid elements required for general use. Hence, the greater the necessity for rapid supply of solid material, the more liquid is removed by perspiration or by the formation of urine, so that new fluid in the shape of chyme or chyle may be introduced into the blood-vessels without unduly distending them.

THE BLADDER is the hollow sac in which the urine is accumulated, as it is secreted by the kidneys, to prevent the necessity which would otherwise be felt for the continual passage of urine.

IN THREE VARIOUS WAYS the blood is nourished and depurated, receiving its additional supplies—first, from the general absorbents; secondly, from the lacteals through the thoracic duct conveying chyle; thirdly, direct from the internal surface of the stomach and small intestines, through the veins, whose contents are conveyed through the liver, and depurated by the lungs, the liver, the kidneys, and the skin. The supplies, in the first place, are all derived from the food, which is digested by the stomach, aided by the bile and pancreatic juice, and converted into chyle, which is absorbed into the blood.

THE ARTICLES OF FOOD which are most adapted to support man, as well as the dog and horse, in a high state of health and energy, are nearly identical in ultimate composition, though somewhat different as they appear to our general senses. In each case food is required for four different purposes—first, for the building up of the machine; secondly, to supply the loss occasioned by its constant tendency to decay, even when in a state of repose; thirdly, to make up for the waste occasioned by wear and tear of the muscular system; and, fourthly, to supply the materials for the heat-producing process. Now these processes are differently carried on, according to the age and habits of the individual; thus, the young animal will call upon the first division far more than the adult, and will, consequently consume much more food; whilst the very old one will be able to sustain life in a state of rest, with little or no demand for any supply but the second and last. If proper food is not supplied to the growing young animal his frame is imperfectly nourished, and he not only is stunted in size, but his growth is not in a proper proportion of parts, and he is unsightly and awkward. The same takes place from overfeeding, when a redundancy seldom, is met with equally in all the various proportions, but rather in some one or two, which are exaggerated to an undue degree, and completely overpower their adjacent members. Thus, fat is stored up in enormous masses in the adult animal; and though it is capable of being afterwards withdrawn, yet it often has in the meantime led to the absorption and loss of those parts upon which it has been lying.

In estimating the value of the various aliments, therefore, the age and the habits must always be taken into consideration, and when this is done it will be found that saccharine and albuminous elements will be required for young animals, rather than those loaded with fibrine; whilst in the adult period this element is required in large quantities; and in old age, oily or starchy compounds, which are full of carbon, and support combustion. Sugar, there is reason to believe, is very readily admitted into the circulation, and supports the process of respiration well—hence its use to young animals. In omnivorous animals, like man and the dog, a mixture of substances containing nitrogen, with others free from it, is the best kind of food; and this is met with in flesh and farinaceous food, together with the saccharine fruits of the earth. But wheaten bread contains the same elements, and upon it either the man or the dog, or even the horse, can be sustained in good health, if accustomed to it from an early stage. With the addition of an animal oil, it will at all times serve for a permanent diet; and in a low temperature will scarcely be sufficient without it, or some fermented liquor in its place. But if violent exercise is taken, flesh should be added, in the case of man or the dog; or in the case of the horse, a large proportion of corn, with, at the same time, *well fermented hay*, in which sugar is thoroughly developed. Rice and potatoes, together with sago, and other articles mostly made up of starch, are chiefly beneficial in supporting respiration, and effect comparatively little towards the repair of the muscular tissues, which are composed in great measure of nitrogen.

Another important consideration in supplying food is the change which is required in its nature, few animals being capable of carrying on digestion of the same materials from week to week without suffering loss of health. Thus, cattle must be moved from one pasture to another; and the horse, after a time, must have a change of food from corn and hay to green food or carrots, or his stomach is sure to suffer. In a state of nature instinct prompts to these changes; and even in a half-artificial condition the hare will travel for miles to obtain what she wants, although to all appearance she has it close to her own haunt.

But these organic substances are not the only ones required by the system; there are also inorganic matters which enter into the composition of the frame, and which must be obtained with the food. *Salt* affords by its decomposition the muriatic acid which is concerned in the digestive process, and the soda of the bile. It is also an important constituent of the serum of the blood, preventing it from being decomposed. *Phosphorus* enters largely into the composition of bone and tissue. *Sulphur*, again, exists in small quantities; and *lime* is abundantly required. *Iron*, also, must be obtained, because its presence is important to the due formation of the red corpuscles. These substances are all obtained from our ordinary food. Salt is abundant in flesh and milk, but it should be supplied to herbivorous animals, like the horse, in addition to his food. Lime is abundant in vegetable seeds, like wheat and oats, and in the grasses; and if these are supplied to the horse he will develop bone in a sufficient quantity.

SECT. 8.—THE ORGANS OF REPRODUCTION

These are the same, or very nearly so, in all the three subjects under examination, each possessing the same male and female organs. The male are only necessary for the elaboration of the semen, and for transmitting it into the uterus of the female; but her part consists in preparing an ovum in the ovarium, in transmitting it safely to the uterus, and in then attaching it to the walls of that organ, and nourishing it for a stated period till birth takes place. This subject has been touched on in page 551, and a more elaborate discussion is scarcely suited to a book like the present.

SECT. 9.—THE ORGANS OF SENSE

In all the three creatures we are now examining the same organs of sense exist, but with varying degrees of acuteness. In man the sense of touch and the eyesight are perhaps more acute than in either the horse or dog; but in the dog the sense of smell is far beyond that of man or the horse; and in the last-named animal the hearing is particularly acute. But, anatomically, these organs differ little, each having the same parts, though varying slightly in detail; as in the shape of the pupil of the eye, which in the horse is oblong horizontally, whilst in the dog and in man it is perfectly circular. The horse also possesses a peculiar structure within the eye, the *tapetum lucidum*, of a lustrous green colour, by which he is enabled to see objects in comparative darkness, and especially under his feet. The external ear also differs in all, but the internal parts of this organ are very similar. The nerves supplying the nose are developed in the dog in a high degree, as are those distributed to the ends of the fingers in man, and as a consequence, these organs are endowed with an extra degree of sensitiveness. The compass of this book, however, will not allow of a full examination of the detail of parts which make up those beautiful organs, the eye and ear.

SECT. 10.—THE SKIN, AND GENERAL CELLULAR MEMBRANE

ALL THE PARTS OF THE BODY are wrapped up first of all in a packing of cellular membrane, which attaches the various muscles, vessels, nerves, and bones intimately together, yet with a power of gliding upon each other which is necessary to their several functions. This is the structure which is blown up in the dead calf, and which consists of a series of cells communicating with each other throughout the body, and therefore capable of being filled by one or two openings made by the butcher, and inflated by him by means of a pipe passed into them. In these cells fat is deposited and stored up for use, and when wanted it is re-absorbed from them, and carried off into the blood to be converted into other needful materials, or used for the purposes of respiration, for which its carbon is eminently calculated. The skin, again, covers and guards all the parts, and keeps them warm and protected from slight injuries. It is pierced by minute openings, through which the sweat is distilled, and also by oil-tubes, which lubricate its surface and keep the hair with which it is more or less covered in a state fit to encounter the watery fluid which rain or flood presents to it. The skin is a highly elastic and yielding, yet tough investment, which will submit to great stretching before it gives way, and is so beautifully adapted to the varying conditions of the animal frame that it fits the lean racehorse as closely as the pampered denizen of the stud.

THE HAIR is a dead matter secreted by certain bulbous glands, which, as they form it, push it through the skin, being in close contact with its inner surface, and protected by it. The hair of man is not regularly shed; but in the dog and horse it grows longer and coarser in the winter than in the summer, and is consequently shed to provide for this necessity of their exposed condition. This takes place in the spring and autumn, and is strongly marked in the horse, whose coat is completely changed in the spring, and partially so in the autumn; and less so in the dog, who only changes his once in a year, and is not provided with one in the winter much longer than in the summer, but has a slight increase of growth added to that which has existed during the warm months. The colour of the hair varies in all; but is confined to black, brown, dusky-red, and white, or some mixture of these—as mottled-grey, iron-grey, roan, strawberry, pie, skewbald, brindle, black-and-tan, dun, and cream-colour.

THE NAILS AND HOOFS are appendages to the skin, and they are also dead matter, secreted much in the same way. Both are composed of a horny matter, elastic, firm, and capable of bearing great friction. The nails of the dog and the hoof of the horse completely surround the bone upon which they are moulded, and have the vascular structure which secretes them lying between it and them. In man, on the other hand, the nail only covers one-half of the tips of his fingers, because a soft pulpy end is wanted for the organ of touch.

Printed in Great Britain
by Amazon